MASTERING THE GLYCEMIC DIET

A Comprehensive Guide to Low-GI Eating for Weight Loss and Wellness

Adams .U. Morris

TABLE OF CONTENTS

CHAPTER 1

Introduction to the Glycemic Diet

In today's fast-paced world, health and nutrition have become paramount concerns. We're bombarded with various diets, each promising better health and a slimmer waistline. Among these diets, the Glycemic Diet has gained significant attention for its potential to not only help us shed those unwanted pounds but also improve overall health. But before we dive into the specifics of the

Glycemic Diet, let's embark on a journey to understand the fundamentals.

The Mystery of Blood Sugar

To unravel the Glycemic Diet, we need to start by cracking the code of blood sugar. Blood sugar, also known as blood glucose, is essentially the sugar present in your bloodstream. It's the body's primary source of energy, and it comes from the carbohydrates we consume in our diet.

Here's where things get interesting. When we eat carbohydrates, our body breaks them down into glucose, which enters our bloodstream. This surge in blood sugar levels triggers the release of insulin, a hormone produced by the pancreas. Insulin's job is to help cells absorb glucose from the bloodstream so that it can be used for energy or stored for later.

Now, here's the twist: some carbohydrates cause a rapid and sharp increase in blood sugar levels, while others lead to a slow and steady rise. This is where the Glycemic Diet comes into play.

The Glycemic Index (GI): The Key Player

Enter the Glycemic Index (GI). The GI is a scale that ranks carbohydrates based on their effect on blood sugar levels. Foods with a high GI are rapidly digested and cause a quick spike in blood sugar, while those with a low GI are digested more slowly, leading to a gradual and sustained release of glucose into the bloodstream.

The GI scale ranges from 0 to 100, with pure glucose set as 100, representing the fastest and highest spike in blood sugar. Foods with a GI below 55 are considered low, those between 56 and 69 are moderate, and those above 70 are high.

The Glycemic Load (GL): Adding a Dimension

But wait, there's more to the story. While the GI is a valuable tool, it doesn't account for portion size. That's where the Glycemic Load (GL) steps in. GL takes both the GI and the quantity of carbohydrates into consideration. It gives you a more realistic picture of how a particular food will affect your blood sugar.

For instance, watermelon has a high GI, but it contains very few carbohydrates per serving. So, its GL is relatively low, meaning it won't cause a significant spike in blood sugar unless you eat an enormous amount.

The Science Behind It All

Now, you might wonder why we should care about all of this. Well, here's the crux of the matter: rapid and frequent spikes in blood sugar can wreak havoc on our health. It can lead to a host of problems, including:

1. **Energy Rollercoaster**: High GI foods can cause a rapid increase in energy

followed by a crash, leaving you feeling tired and irritable.

2. **Weight Gain**: The insulin response triggered by high GI foods can promote fat storage, making it difficult to lose weight.

3. **Type 2 Diabetes**: Over time, consistently high blood sugar levels can lead to insulin resistance, a key factor in the development of type 2 diabetes.

4. **Heart Health**: Elevated blood sugar is linked to an increased risk of heart disease.

5. **Hunger and Overeating**: High GI foods often fail to provide a feeling of fullness, leading to overeating and weight gain.

The Glycemic Diet Solution

So, what does the Glycemic Diet propose to do? It advocates for a shift towards consuming foods with a lower GI and GL. By doing this, you can:

1. **Stabilize Blood Sugar**: Opting for low GI foods helps prevent those drastic spikes and crashes in blood sugar levels. This results in a

more consistent and sustainable energy supply throughout the day.

2. **Aid in Weight Management**: A diet that focuses on low GI foods can help with weight management because it promotes a feeling of fullness, making it easier to control your calorie intake.

3. **Reduce Diabetes Risk**: For those at risk of or dealing with type 2 diabetes, a Glycemic Diet can be a powerful tool for better blood sugar control.

4. **Enhance Heart Health**: A diet that minimizes high GI foods can contribute to a healthier heart by reducing the risk of heart disease.

The Versatility of the Glycemic Diet

One of the remarkable aspects of the Glycemic Diet is its versatility. It's not a one-size-fits-all approach. Whether you're an athlete looking for sustained energy, a mom-to-be concerned about gestational diabetes, or someone simply striving for better health, the Glycemic Diet can be adapted to suit your specific needs.

What's Next?

In this introductory chapter, we've laid the foundation for our exploration of the Glycemic Diet. We've learned that the Glycemic Index and Glycemic Load are the keys to understanding how different carbohydrates affect our blood sugar levels. We've also seen the potential benefits of adopting a diet that emphasizes low GI and low GL foods, from stable energy levels to better weight management and reduced health risks.

As we move forward in this book, we'll delve deeper into the specifics of the Glycemic Diet. We'll explore various food groups, meal planning, and strategies to make this diet work for you. Whether you're a newcomer to the concept or someone seeking to refine their approach, this journey promises to be both enlightening and rewarding. Welcome to the world of the Glycemic Diet, where knowledge is the first step towards a healthier, happier you.

CHAPTER 2

Understanding Carbohydrates

Now that we've grasped the basics of blood sugar and the Glycemic Index in Chapter 1, it's time to take a closer look at the unsung heroes and sometimes misunderstood culprits of the Glycemic Diet – carbohydrates.

Carbohydrates: The Body's Energy Source

Carbohydrates, often referred to as "carbs," are one of the three macronutrients, alongside protein and fat. They are a primary source of energy for our bodies. Picture them as the fuel that powers your car; they keep you running.

Types of Carbohydrates: Simple vs. Complex

Not all carbs are created equal. Carbohydrates can be broadly categorized into two main types: simple and complex.

1. **Simple Carbohydrates**: These are made up of one or two sugar units, making them easy to digest and absorb quickly into the

bloodstream. Simple carbs are often found in foods like table sugar, sugary snacks, and sweetened beverages. They're the culprits behind those rapid blood sugar spikes we want to avoid.

2. **Complex Carbohydrates**: In contrast, complex carbs consist of longer chains of sugar molecules. These chains take more time and energy to break down, leading to a gradual and steady release of glucose into the bloodstream. Complex carbs are abundant in foods

like whole grains, vegetables, and legumes.

The Glycemic Response: Simple vs. Complex Carbs

Here's where the Glycemic Index (GI) comes into play. It helps us understand how different carbs affect our blood sugar levels. Simple carbs, with their short sugar chains, tend to have high GI values, causing that rapid spike in blood sugar.

On the other hand, complex carbs, with their longer chains, usually have low to moderate GI values. This means they're digested more slowly, providing a sustained source of energy without the rollercoaster effect on blood sugar.

Fiber: The Carb's Sidekick

Now, let's introduce a sidekick in the carbohydrate world – fiber. Fiber is a type of carbohydrate that the body can't digest. It's found in plant-based foods like fruits, vegetables, whole grains, nuts, and seeds. Fiber plays a crucial role in the Glycemic Diet for several reasons:

1. **Slowing Digestion**: Fiber adds bulk to your meals, slowing down the digestion

and absorption of carbohydrates. This helps prevent rapid blood sugar spikes.

2. **Promoting Fullness**: Foods high in fiber are often more filling, which can help with portion control and weight management.

3. **Heart Health**: Soluble fiber, in particular, has been shown to lower cholesterol levels, benefiting heart health.

The Glycemic Index of Carbohydrate Sources

Let's break down some common sources of carbohydrates and their GI values:

1. **Whole Grains**: Whole grains like oats, quinoa, and brown rice typically have low to moderate GI values. They're excellent choices for sustained energy.

2. **Starchy Vegetables**: Vegetables like sweet potatoes, corn, and peas fall into the moderate GI range. They provide valuable nutrients alongside energy.

3. **Legumes**: Beans, lentils, and chickpeas are

champions of the low GI category. They're rich in fiber and protein, making them a stable energy source.

4. **Fruits**: Fruits can vary widely in their GI values. Berries and apples have low GI values, while watermelon and pineapple have higher GIs.

5. **Refined Carbs**: Foods made from refined grains, like white bread and most breakfast cereals, often have high GI values. These are best consumed in moderation.

Balancing Carbohydrates in Your Diet

Now, you might be thinking, "Do I need to completely eliminate high-GI carbs?" The answer is no. The Glycemic Diet isn't about exclusion; it's about balance and making informed choices.

Here are some practical tips for balancing carbohydrates in your diet:

1. **Choose Whole Grains**: Opt for whole grain bread, pasta, and rice instead of their refined counterparts.

These choices offer more fiber and nutrients.

2. **Mind Your Portions**: Be mindful of portion sizes, especially when it comes to higher GI foods. A small serving of white rice alongside a larger portion of vegetables can help balance the meal.

3. **Combine Foods Wisely**: Combining high-GI foods with sources of protein, healthy fats, and fiber can slow down the absorption of glucose. For example, have almond butter with your toast instead of jam.

4. **Snack Smart**: When snacking, reach for options like Greek yogurt, nuts, or vegetables with hummus to keep your energy levels steady.

5. **Explore Low-GI Alternatives**: Discover lower GI alternatives to your favorite foods. For instance, try cauliflower rice instead of white rice for a lower-GI side dish.

The Power of Knowledge

Understanding carbohydrates and how they affect your blood sugar is a cornerstone of the Glycemic

Diet. Armed with this knowledge, you're better equipped to make informed choices about what you eat. It's not about vilifying carbs but rather choosing them wisely to support stable energy levels, weight management, and overall health.

As we journey through this book, we'll delve deeper into practical strategies for implementing the Glycemic Diet in your daily life. We'll explore meal planning, recipes, and ways to navigate various dietary needs and preferences while still reaping the benefits of this approach.

In the end, it's about enjoying a well-balanced diet that works for you, allowing you to savor the flavors of life without sacrificing your health and well-being. So, let's continue this voyage of discovery and transformation together, one carbohydrate at a time.

CHAPTER 3

The Glycemic Index Explained

In Chapter 2, we delved into the world of carbohydrates, distinguishing between simple and complex carbs and introducing the concept of fiber. Now, it's time to dive deeper into one of the pivotal elements of the Glycemic Diet - the Glycemic Index (GI).

The Glycemic Index: A Refresher

To understand this chapter fully, let's start with a quick refresher. The Glycemic Index (GI) is a numerical scale that ranks carbohydrates based on their impact on blood sugar levels. Foods with a high GI are quickly digested and cause rapid spikes in blood sugar, while those with a low GI are digested more slowly, leading to a gradual and sustained release of glucose into the bloodstream.

The GI scale ranges from 0 to 100, with pure glucose serving as the reference point at 100. Any food with a GI below 55 is considered low, while those between 56 and 69 are moderate, and anything above 70 is considered high.

How GI Values Are Determined

The GI value of a food is determined through controlled scientific testing. Here's the basic process:

1. **Test Subjects**: A group of healthy individuals is selected as test subjects.

2. **Carb Consumption**: Each subject consumes a measured amount of the test food, typically providing 50

grams of carbohydrates. This amount is chosen because it's roughly equivalent across different foods.

3. **Blood Sugar Monitoring**: Over the next few hours, researchers regularly draw blood from the subjects to measure their blood sugar levels. These measurements create a curve that shows how quickly and to what extent blood sugar rises after eating the test food.

4. **Comparative Analysis**: The researchers then compare the blood sugar curve of the test food to that

of pure glucose. The area under the curve is calculated for both. If the test food's curve is similar to that of glucose, it gets a high GI value. If it's significantly different, it gets a lower GI value.

Why Does the Glycemic Index Matter?

Now, let's get to the heart of the matter. Why should you care about the GI of the foods you eat? There are several reasons:

Blood Sugar Control: For those concerned about blood sugar levels, especially individuals with diabetes or prediabetes, understanding the GI of foods can help manage their condition. Low-GI foods lead to slower, steadier blood sugar responses, which can be crucial for those who need to avoid spikes and crashes.

Energy Levels: Foods with a lower GI provide a more sustained source of energy. They can help prevent the energy highs and lows associated with high-GI meals, keeping you alert and focused throughout the day.

Weight Management: The Glycemic Diet's emphasis on low-

GI foods can aid in weight management. High-GI foods can trigger hunger and cravings shortly after eating, leading to overconsumption. Low-GI foods tend to keep you feeling full for longer, which can help control your calorie intake.

Heart Health: Diets rich in low-GI foods have been associated with improved heart health. They can help lower LDL ("bad") cholesterol levels and reduce the risk of heart disease.

Athletic Performance: Athletes often utilize the GI to optimize their energy levels during training and competition. Low-GI foods can provide sustained energy, which is essential for endurance sports.

The Practical Side of GI

While understanding the GI of foods is valuable, applying it to your daily life can seem daunting. Here are some practical considerations:

1. **Mixed Meals**: In real-life meals, foods are rarely consumed in isolation. Combining high-GI and low-GI foods can moderate the overall GI of a meal. For

example, adding a protein source or healthy fats to high-GI rice can slow its digestion.

2. **Individual Variations**: It's important to note that the GI can vary between individuals and even in the same individual under different circumstances. Factors like food ripeness, cooking methods, and genetics can influence how your body responds to a particular food.

3. **Use as a Guide**: The GI is a valuable guide, but it doesn't have to dictate your entire

diet. Consider it a tool in your nutritional toolbox. Focus on incorporating more low-GI foods rather than rigidly avoiding all high-GI options.

Misconceptions and Criticisms of the GI

While the GI has gained popularity and recognition, it's not without its critics and misconceptions. Here are a few points to keep in mind:

1. **Variability**: As mentioned earlier, the GI of a food can vary due to several factors.

This variability has led some to question the GI's reliability as a practical guide for meal planning.

2. **Focus on Single Foods**: GI values are typically determined for individual foods, not for entire meals. In reality, meals are composed of multiple foods, and the overall GI of a meal can differ from the GI of its individual components.

3. **Complexity**: Calculating the GI of a meal can be complex, especially when considering various factors and combinations. This

complexity can make it challenging to apply the GI effectively in everyday life.

The Bottom Line

In this chapter, we've explored the Glycemic Index in depth. It's a valuable tool for understanding how different carbohydrates affect our blood sugar levels. By incorporating more low-GI foods into your diet and being mindful of portion sizes, you can work towards stable blood sugar levels, improved energy, and better overall health.

In the upcoming chapters of this book, we'll move beyond theory and explore practical strategies for implementing the Glycemic Diet in your daily life. We'll discuss meal planning, offer delicious recipes, and provide guidance on how to adapt this approach to various dietary needs and preferences.

So, as you continue on this journey towards better health through the Glycemic Diet, remember that knowledge is your ally. Armed with an understanding of the GI, you have the power to make informed choices that can positively impact your well-being.

CHAPTER 4

Practical Tips for a Low GI Diet

Now that we've established a solid foundation about carbohydrates and the Glycemic Index (GI) in the previous chapters, it's time to roll up our sleeves and get practical. In Chapter 4, we'll delve into the nitty-gritty of adopting a low GI diet. This chapter is all about turning knowledge into action.

1. Grocery Shopping for Success

Your journey towards a low GI diet begins at the grocery store. Here are some tips to help you make smart choices in the aisles:

- **Read Labels**: Check the nutritional labels on packaged foods. Look for the GI value if it's available. Pay attention to total carbohydrates, fiber, and added sugars.

- **Choose Whole Foods**: Focus on the perimeter of the store, where you'll find fresh produce, lean proteins, and whole grains. These are the building blocks of a low GI diet.

- **Variety Matters**: Embrace variety in your shopping cart. The more colorful your fruits and vegetables, the wider the range of nutrients you'll consume.

- **Buy Legumes**: Load up on legumes like beans, lentils, and chickpeas. They're low GI, high in protein and fiber, making them superstars in the low GI world.

- **Opt for Whole Grains**: When it comes to grains, choose whole grains like brown rice, whole wheat pasta, and oats. They're lower GI options compared to their refined counterparts.

2. Cooking and Meal Preparation Techniques

Once you've filled your pantry and fridge with low GI ingredients, it's time to put them to good use in the kitchen. Here are some cooking and meal preparation techniques to keep in mind:

- **Cooking Methods**: Steaming, boiling, and baking are great cooking methods for preserving the low GI of foods. Avoid frying, as it can increase the GI of some foods.

- **Pair with Protein**: Combine carbohydrates with protein sources like chicken, fish, tofu, or legumes. This slows down digestion and helps stabilize blood sugar.

- **Add Healthy Fats**: Incorporate healthy fats like olive oil, avocado, and nuts into your meals. They add flavor and can further slow the absorption of glucose.

- **Mindful Portions**: Be aware of portion sizes. Even low GI foods can impact blood sugar if consumed in excess. Use measuring cups and kitchen scales to help with portion control.

3. Portion Control and Mindful Eating

Portion control is a fundamental aspect of managing the GI of your meals. Here are some strategies to help you eat mindfully:

- **Use Smaller Plates**: Serve meals on smaller plates to help control portion sizes. Research shows that this simple trick can prevent overeating.

- **Chew Slowly**: Take your time to chew each bite thoroughly. Eating slowly gives your body more time to register fullness, reducing the likelihood of overeating.

- **Practice Mindful Eating**: Pay attention to your body's hunger and fullness cues. Eat when you're hungry, and stop when you're satisfied, not stuffed.

- **Avoid Distractions**: Eating in front of the TV or computer can lead to mindless overeating. Try to eat at a designated dining area without distractions.

4. Building Balanced Low GI Meals

Creating balanced, low GI meals is at the heart of this diet. Here's a simple formula to guide your meal planning:

- **Lean Protein**: Include a source of lean protein like chicken, fish, tofu, or beans. Protein helps keep you full and stabilizes blood sugar.
- **Fiber-Rich Carbs**: Incorporate plenty of vegetables and whole grains into your meals. These provide fiber, vitamins, and

minerals while keeping the GI low.

- **Healthy Fats**: Add a touch of healthy fats, such as olive oil, avocado, or nuts. They enhance the flavor and satisfaction of your meals.

- **Limit Sugar**: Minimize added sugars and sugary beverages. These can cause rapid blood sugar spikes.

- **Hydration**: Stay hydrated with water or herbal teas. Dehydration can sometimes be mistaken for hunger.

5. Snacking Smart

Snacking can be an ally or an adversary when it comes to low GI eating. Here's how to make it work for you:

- **Plan Your Snacks**: Pre-plan your snacks so that you're not reaching for high-GI options when hunger strikes.

- **Go for Protein**: Opt for protein-rich snacks like Greek yogurt, cheese, or a handful of almonds. These can help maintain blood sugar stability between meals.

- **Portion Control**: Use small containers or zip-lock bags to portion out snacks. This prevents mindless munching.

- **Fruits and Veggies**: Keep cut-up fruits and veggies in the fridge for quick, low-GI snack options.

6. Dining Out Mindfully

Eating out doesn't have to derail your low GI efforts. Here's how to make informed choices at restaurants:

- **Check Menus Online**: Many restaurants now

provide nutrition information on their websites. Take a look before you go to plan your order.

- **Ask Questions**: Don't hesitate to ask your server about how dishes are prepared. Request modifications to make your meal lower GI if needed.

- **Share Dishes**: Consider sharing high-GI dishes with friends or family to enjoy a taste without overindulging.

- **Skip Sugary Drinks**: Opt for water or unsweetened beverages instead of sugary sodas or cocktails.

7. Be Patient and Persistent

Remember, adopting a low GI diet is a lifestyle change, not a quick fix. It may take time to see noticeable changes in your energy levels, weight, or blood sugar control. Be patient with yourself and stay persistent.

8. Experiment and Enjoy

Lastly, don't forget to have fun with your low GI journey. Experiment with new recipes, ingredients, and cooking techniques. Explore the world of flavors that low GI foods have to offer. This diet isn't about deprivation; it's about making delicious and nutritious choices that benefit your health.

In Chapter 5, we'll explore how the Glycemic Diet can be a valuable tool for weight management. We'll delve into the science behind how a low GI diet can aid in shedding pounds and maintaining a healthy weight. So, stay tuned, and keep up the good work on your low GI adventure!

CHAPTER 5

Glycemic Diet and Weight Management

In the previous chapters, we've laid the groundwork for understanding the Glycemic Diet, from carbohydrates and the Glycemic Index to practical tips for incorporating low-GI foods into your daily life. Now, let's delve into a topic that often sparks considerable interest - how the Glycemic Diet can play a pivotal role in weight management.

The Weight Management Conundrum

Weight management is a journey that millions of people embark on every day. In a world filled with fad diets and trendy weight loss programs, it's crucial to focus on approaches that are sustainable, effective, and, most importantly, good for your long-term health. This is where the Glycemic Diet shines.

Why Does the Glycemic Diet Matter for Weight Management?

To understand why the Glycemic Diet is a powerful tool for weight management, we need to revisit the concept of the Glycemic Index (GI). As we've learned, the GI ranks carbohydrates based on how quickly they affect blood sugar levels. Low-GI foods are digested slowly, leading to gradual and sustained increases in blood sugar.

Now, consider the impact of high-GI foods on your weight management journey:

1. **Blood Sugar Rollercoaster**: When you consume high-GI foods, your blood sugar levels spike

quickly, leading to a surge in energy. However, this spike is often followed by a crash, leaving you feeling tired, irritable, and craving more sugary or high-GI foods to regain energy.

2. **Increased Appetite**: This blood sugar rollercoaster can trigger hunger pangs and cravings for more carbohydrates, particularly sugary and starchy options. You're more likely to overeat when you're constantly battling cravings.

3. **Insulin and Fat Storage**: High-GI foods prompt your

pancreas to release a surge of insulin to shuttle glucose into your cells. However, this insulin response can also promote fat storage. Excess glucose in your bloodstream gets converted and stored as fat.

4. **Vicious Cycle**: The cycle of energy spikes, crashes, and cravings can become a vicious cycle that makes it difficult to control your calorie intake, ultimately leading to weight gain.

Now, let's see how a low-GI approach can counter these challenges:

Steady Energy Levels: Low-GI foods are digested slowly and lead to a gradual and sustained increase in blood sugar. This provides you with a more stable and prolonged source of energy, reducing the temptation to reach for high-GI snacks.

Fullness and Satisfaction: Low-GI foods, often high in fiber and protein, promote a feeling of fullness and satiety. You're less likely to overeat or experience intense hunger shortly after a meal.

Better Blood Sugar Control: For individuals with insulin resistance or prediabetes, a low-GI diet can help improve blood sugar control, reducing the risk of further weight gain.

Reduced Cravings: Low-GI meals can help stabilize blood sugar levels, reducing the frequency and intensity of cravings for high-GI, sugary snacks.

Weight Loss with the Glycemic Diet

Numerous studies have explored the relationship between the Glycemic Diet and weight loss. While individual results can vary, here are some key findings:

1. **Gradual Weight Loss**: The gradual and sustainable nature of low-GI foods can contribute to steady, long-term weight loss. This approach focuses on lifestyle changes rather than quick fixes.

2. **Improved Fat Loss**: Some research suggests that low-GI diets may promote fat loss while preserving lean

muscle mass. This is particularly beneficial because maintaining muscle can boost metabolism.

3. **Appetite Control**: Low-GI meals tend to keep you feeling full for longer periods. This can lead to reduced calorie intake throughout the day, supporting weight loss efforts.

4. **Blood Sugar Regulation**: Individuals with diabetes or insulin resistance may experience improved blood sugar control when following a low-GI diet. This can lead

to better weight management.

5. **Sustainable Approach**: Unlike some restrictive diets, the Glycemic Diet is sustainable in the long term. It encourages a balanced and varied diet, making it more likely for people to stick with it.

Practical Strategies for Weight Management with the Glycemic Diet

Implementing a low-GI approach for weight management doesn't have to be complex or daunting.

Here are some practical strategies to help you on your journey:

1. Balanced Meals: Build balanced meals that include lean protein, fiber-rich carbohydrates (such as vegetables and whole grains), and healthy fats. This combination helps control hunger and stabilize blood sugar.

2. Portion Control: Be mindful of portion sizes, even when eating low-GI foods. Overeating can still lead to weight gain, so practice moderation.

3. Snack Smart: Choose low-GI snacks like Greek yogurt, nuts, or raw vegetables with hummus to keep energy levels steady between meals.

4. Hydration: Drink plenty of water throughout the day. Sometimes, thirst is mistaken for hunger, leading to unnecessary snacking.

5. Consistency: Consistency is key. Aim to make low-GI eating a habit rather than a short-term solution. Sustainable changes yield long-term results.

6. Exercise: Combine a low-GI diet with regular physical activity for maximum benefits. Exercise helps burn calories, build lean muscle, and improve overall health.

7. Seek Support: Consider seeking support from a registered dietitian or nutritionist who can provide personalized guidance and help you navigate your weight management journey.

8. Mindfulness: Pay attention to your body's hunger and fullness cues. Eating mindfully can prevent overeating and emotional eating.

9. Be Patient and Realistic: Weight management takes time, and progress may be gradual. Set realistic goals and celebrate your achievements along the way.

10. Enjoy the Journey: Embrace the variety and flavors that low-GI foods offer. Eating should be a pleasurable experience, and there are countless delicious low-GI recipes to explore.

The Glycemic Diet's Holistic Approach

What sets the Glycemic Diet apart from many other weight loss plans is its holistic approach. It's not just about shedding pounds; it's about improving overall health and well-being. By focusing on stable blood sugar levels, you're not only working towards a healthy weight, but you're also reducing the risk of chronic diseases like type 2 diabetes and heart disease.

In the upcoming chapters, we'll continue our exploration of the Glycemic Diet, touching on its applications in blood sugar control, heart health, and catering to special dietary needs. Remember, this journey is not just about losing weight; it's about achieving and maintaining a balanced, vibrant life through

informed choices and sustainable
habits.

CHAPTER 6

Glycemic Diet and Blood Sugar Control

Welcome to Chapter 6 of our journey through the Glycemic Diet. We've already covered a lot of ground, from understanding carbohydrates and the Glycemic Index to practical tips for meal planning and weight management. Now, it's time to dive into a critical aspect of this diet – how it can help manage blood sugar levels, especially for individuals with diabetes or prediabetes.

The Diabetes Epidemic

Diabetes is a growing global health concern. It's a condition characterized by high blood sugar levels resulting from the body's inability to effectively use or produce insulin, the hormone responsible for regulating blood sugar. There are two main types of diabetes:

1. **Type 1 Diabetes**: This autoimmune condition typically develops in childhood or adolescence. People with type 1 diabetes require lifelong insulin

therapy because their bodies don't produce insulin.

2. **Type 2 Diabetes**: This form of diabetes is more common and often develops later in life. It's associated with insulin resistance, where the body's cells don't respond effectively to insulin, and eventually, the pancreas can't produce enough insulin to maintain normal blood sugar levels.

Prediabetes is a precursor to type 2 diabetes, characterized by elevated blood sugar levels that aren't yet in the diabetic range. If left unchecked, prediabetes can progress to type 2 diabetes.

The Role of the Glycemic Diet in Blood Sugar Control

The Glycemic Diet is particularly relevant for individuals with diabetes and prediabetes because it focuses on the quality of carbohydrates consumed. By emphasizing low-GI foods, this diet helps prevent rapid spikes in blood sugar levels, which is crucial for those who need to manage their condition effectively.

Here's how the Glycemic Diet supports blood sugar control:

1. Stabilizing Blood Sugar Levels

Low-GI foods are digested slowly, leading to a gradual and sustained increase in blood sugar. This helps prevent the rapid and sometimes dangerous spikes in blood sugar that can occur after consuming high-GI foods.

For individuals with diabetes, these blood sugar spikes can be problematic because their bodies may struggle to produce enough insulin to counteract them. By choosing low-GI options, they can maintain more stable blood sugar levels throughout the day.

2. Reducing Insulin Demand

The Glycemic Diet's focus on low-GI foods can also reduce the demand for insulin. In type 2 diabetes, insulin resistance means that cells don't respond well to insulin, and the pancreas has to produce more to compensate. By consuming low-GI foods, which require less insulin for processing, the burden on the pancreas is eased.

3. Supporting Weight Management

Weight management is closely linked to blood sugar control,

especially in type 2 diabetes and prediabetes. Excess body weight can contribute to insulin resistance, making blood sugar management more challenging.

The Glycemic Diet's emphasis on whole, low-GI foods can aid in weight loss and weight maintenance. By keeping you full and satisfied, it helps control calorie intake, which is essential for managing body weight.

4. Aiding in Medication Management

For individuals with diabetes who require medication or insulin therapy, a low-GI diet can complement their treatment. By helping maintain stable blood sugar levels, it can reduce the risk of hypoglycemia (low blood sugar) and minimize the need for medication adjustments.

5. Improving Long-Term Health

Diabetes management is not just about controlling blood sugar levels today; it's also about preventing complications in the long term. Elevated blood sugar levels can damage blood vessels, nerves, and organs over time, leading to serious health issues like heart disease, kidney disease, and nerve damage.

The Glycemic Diet's potential to improve blood sugar control can contribute to better long-term health outcomes by reducing the risk of these complications.

Practical Strategies for Blood Sugar Control with the Glycemic Diet

Now, let's explore some practical strategies for incorporating the Glycemic Diet into your daily life for effective blood sugar control:

1. **Carb Counting**: Learn to count carbohydrates accurately.

This helps individuals with diabetes match their insulin or medication doses to their carbohydrate intake. While the Glycemic Diet focuses on low-GI foods, the total amount of carbohydrates still matters.

2. Portion Control: Be mindful of portion sizes. Even low-GI foods can affect blood sugar when consumed in excessive amounts. Use measuring cups and scales to help with portion control.

3. Balanced Meals: Create balanced meals that include lean protein, fiber-rich carbohydrates (such as vegetables and whole grains), and healthy fats. This balance can help stabilize blood sugar levels.

4. Consistency: Consistency in meal timing can help regulate blood sugar. Try to eat meals and snacks at roughly the same times each day.

5. Monitor Blood Sugar: Regularly monitor your blood sugar levels as recommended by your healthcare provider. This helps you understand how your dietary choices impact your blood sugar and allows for necessary adjustments.

6. Be Prepared: Plan your meals and snacks in advance. Having low-GI options readily available can prevent you from reaching for high-GI foods in moments of hunger.

7. Seek Support: If you have diabetes, consider working with a registered dietitian or diabetes educator. They can provide personalized guidance and support in managing your diet.

8. Stay Active: Regular physical activity can improve insulin sensitivity and support blood sugar control. Aim for a combination of aerobic exercise and strength training.

9. Hydrate: Drink plenty of water throughout the day. Dehydration can affect blood sugar levels, so staying hydrated is essential.

10. Medication Management: If you're taking medications or insulin, work closely with your healthcare provider to adjust your treatment plan as needed. Changes in your diet can impact your medication requirements.

11. Be Informed: Stay informed about the Glycemic Index and how it applies to different foods.

Knowledge is your ally in making informed choices.

The Holistic Approach to Health

The Glycemic Diet's focus on blood sugar control isn't just about managing a condition; it's about promoting overall health and well-being. By stabilizing blood sugar levels, individuals with diabetes can reduce the risk of complications and enjoy a higher quality of life.

In the upcoming chapters of this book, we'll continue to explore the diverse applications of the

Glycemic Diet. We'll delve into its role in heart health, its adaptability for various dietary needs, and practical meal planning and recipe ideas. Remember, your health journey is a holistic one, and the Glycemic Diet is a versatile tool to help you along the way.

CHAPTER 7

Glycemic Diet and Heart Health

Welcome to Chapter 7 of our exploration into the Glycemic Diet. In previous chapters, we've covered topics ranging from the fundamentals of the Glycemic Index (GI) to its applications in weight management and blood sugar control. Now, we turn our attention to another crucial aspect of this diet – its role in promoting heart health.

The Link Between Diet and Heart Health

Heart disease remains one of the leading causes of death worldwide. Lifestyle factors, including diet, play a significant role in its development and prevention. The Glycemic Diet offers a dietary approach that can contribute to better heart health in several ways.

Understanding the Glycemic Index and Heart Health

At the heart of the Glycemic Diet is the concept of the Glycemic Index (GI). As a quick recap, the GI ranks carbohydrates based on how quickly they affect blood sugar levels. Low-GI foods are digested slowly, leading to gradual and sustained increases in blood sugar.

So, how does this relate to heart health? Let's break it down:

1. Blood Sugar Control

Blood sugar control isn't just vital for individuals with diabetes; it's also essential for heart health. Elevated blood sugar levels can contribute to inflammation and oxidative stress, which can damage blood vessels and increase the risk of heart disease.

Low-GI foods, which promote stable blood sugar levels, can reduce the risk of these adverse effects. By minimizing blood sugar spikes, they contribute to a healthier vascular system.

2. Weight Management

Maintaining a healthy weight is a cornerstone of heart health. Excess body weight, especially abdominal fat, is associated with an increased risk of heart disease. The Glycemic Diet's focus on whole, low-GI foods supports weight management by helping control calorie intake and reducing the likelihood of overeating.

3. Improved Lipid Profiles

The Glycemic Diet can positively influence lipid profiles. Research has shown that it may help lower levels of low-density lipoprotein (LDL) cholesterol, often referred to as "bad" cholesterol. High LDL cholesterol is a significant risk factor for heart disease.

Low-GI foods, particularly those high in soluble fiber (found in oats, beans, and certain fruits), can contribute to improved cholesterol levels. Soluble fiber binds to cholesterol in the digestive tract, helping to remove it from the body.

4. Reduced Risk of Type 2 Diabetes

Type 2 diabetes is a significant risk factor for heart disease. The Glycemic Diet, by promoting stable blood sugar levels and reducing the risk of type 2 diabetes, indirectly supports heart health. Managing blood sugar is a crucial part of diabetes prevention.

5. Blood Pressure Management

High blood pressure (hypertension) is a well-established risk factor for heart disease. Some research suggests that a low-GI diet may help lower blood pressure, possibly due to its impact on weight management and improved blood sugar control.

Practical Strategies for Heart Health with the Glycemic Diet

Now that we've explored the relationship between the Glycemic Diet and heart health, let's delve into some practical strategies for incorporating this dietary approach into your daily life:

1. Focus on Fiber-Rich Foods

Aim to include plenty of fiber-rich foods in your diet. Fiber helps control cholesterol levels and supports heart health. Good sources of fiber include whole grains, legumes (beans and lentils), vegetables, and fruits.

2. Choose Whole Grains

Opt for whole grains over refined grains. Whole grains like brown rice, whole wheat pasta, and oats are not only lower on the GI but also contain more nutrients and fiber that benefit your heart.

3. Lean Protein Sources

Incorporate lean sources of protein into your meals. Lean meats, poultry, fish, tofu, and legumes are excellent choices.

These protein sources are lower in saturated fat, which can be detrimental to heart health in excess.

4. Healthy Fats

Include healthy fats in your diet. Olive oil, avocados, nuts, and seeds provide heart-healthy monounsaturated and polyunsaturated fats. These fats can help lower LDL cholesterol levels.

5. Limit Saturated and Trans Fats

Minimize saturated and trans fats in your diet. These fats can raise

LDL cholesterol levels and increase the risk of heart disease. Limit your intake of red meat, full-fat dairy products, and processed foods containing trans fats.

6. Mindful Portion Control

Be mindful of portion sizes to manage calorie intake effectively. Even healthy foods can contribute to weight gain if consumed in excess.

7. Stay Hydrated

Drink plenty of water throughout the day. Staying hydrated is essential for overall health, including heart health.

8. Reduce Added Sugars

Limit foods and beverages with added sugars. Sugary foods can contribute to weight gain and negatively impact blood sugar levels, which can affect heart health.

9. Regular Physical Activity

Combine a heart-healthy diet with regular physical activity. Exercise helps maintain a healthy weight, improve lipid profiles, and support overall cardiovascular health.

10. Monitor Your Numbers

If you have risk factors for heart disease, such as high blood pressure or high cholesterol, work with your healthcare provider to monitor and manage these numbers. Regular check-ups and screenings are essential for early intervention.

11. Avoid Processed Foods

Minimize your consumption of processed and highly refined foods, as they often contain hidden sugars and unhealthy fats that can harm heart health.

12. Plan Balanced Meals

Create balanced meals that include a variety of food groups. A well-rounded diet provides essential nutrients and supports overall health.

The Holistic Approach to Heart Health

The Glycemic Diet's impact on heart health exemplifies its holistic approach to well-being. By focusing on the quality of carbohydrates and their effect on blood sugar, this diet benefits not only individuals with diabetes but also those looking to reduce their risk of heart disease.

In the remaining chapters of this book, we'll explore practical meal planning, offer delicious recipes, and discuss how the Glycemic Diet can cater to specific dietary needs and preferences. Remember, your journey to better health encompasses various aspects of your life, and the Glycemic Diet can be a valuable tool in achieving your goals, including maintaining a healthy heart.

CHAPTER 8

Customizing the Glycemic Diet for Your Needs

Welcome to the final chapter of our exploration into the Glycemic Diet. Throughout this journey, we've covered the essentials of this dietary approach, from understanding carbohydrates and the Glycemic Index to its applications in weight management, blood sugar control, and heart health. Now, we reach a pivotal point in your Glycemic Diet adventure – how to tailor this approach to your unique dietary needs and preferences.

One Diet, Many Possibilities

One of the strengths of the Glycemic Diet is its versatility. It's not a one-size-fits-all approach. Instead, it provides a framework that can be customized to suit a wide range of dietary needs and lifestyles. Whether you're a vegetarian, have food allergies, or follow a specific cultural or ethical diet, the Glycemic Diet can be adapted to work for you.

Customizing the Glycemic Diet

Here's how you can customize the Glycemic Diet to meet your specific needs:

1. Vegetarian or Vegan Glycemic Diet

If you're a vegetarian or vegan, you can still follow the Glycemic Diet while excluding animal products. Here's how:

- **Protein Sources**: Replace meat with plant-based protein sources like tofu, tempeh, legumes (beans, lentils, chickpeas), and seitan.

- **Dairy Alternatives**: Choose dairy alternatives like almond milk, soy yogurt, and cashew cheese to replace dairy products.

- **Healthy Fats**: Incorporate plant-based fats like avocado, nuts, seeds, and olive oil.

- **Whole Grains**: Continue to enjoy whole grains such as brown rice, quinoa, and whole wheat pasta.

2. Gluten-Free Glycemic Diet

For those with celiac disease or gluten sensitivity, it's entirely possible to follow a gluten-free Glycemic Diet:

- **Gluten-Free Grains**: Opt for gluten-free grains like rice, quinoa, oats (labeled as gluten-free), and corn.

- **Legumes**: Lean heavily on legumes for protein and fiber.

- **Low-GI Vegetables**: Fill your plate with low-GI vegetables like leafy greens, broccoli, and zucchini.

- **Check Labels**: Be vigilant about checking labels for

gluten-containing ingredients, especially in processed foods.

- **Gluten-Free Baking**: Experiment with gluten-free flours like almond flour, coconut flour, and rice flour in your baking.

3. Paleo Glycemic Diet

The Glycemic Diet can be adapted to align with the principles of the paleo diet, which emphasizes whole foods that our ancestors would have eaten:

- **Lean Proteins**: Focus on lean meats, poultry, and fish.

- **Low-GI Vegetables**: Incorporate non-starchy, low-GI vegetables like leafy greens, cauliflower, and peppers.

- **Healthy Fats**: Enjoy healthy fats from sources like avocado, nuts, seeds, and olive oil.

- **Limit Grains**: Reduce or eliminate grains entirely, including whole grains. Instead, you can occasionally include small amounts of starchy vegetables like sweet potatoes.

- **Fruit in Moderation**: Limit fruit consumption to

lower-GI options like berries and avoid high-GI fruits like watermelon.

- **No Processed Foods**: Strictly avoid processed and refined foods.

4. Mediterranean Glycemic Diet

The Mediterranean diet is renowned for its heart-healthy benefits. You can combine the principles of the Mediterranean diet with the Glycemic Diet:

- **Olive Oil**: Use extra virgin olive oil as your primary source of fat.

- **Fruits and Vegetables**: Incorporate a wide variety of colorful fruits and vegetables.

- **Whole Grains**: Include whole grains like whole wheat bread, pasta, and brown rice in moderation.

- **Lean Proteins**: Choose lean protein sources like fish, poultry, beans, and legumes.

- **Nuts and Seeds**: Enjoy nuts and seeds as snacks and toppings.

- **Wine in Moderation**: If you drink alcohol, consider a

glass of red wine in moderation.

- **Herbs and Spices**: Flavor your dishes with herbs and spices like basil, oregano, and garlic.

5. Low-Lactose Glycemic Diet

If you're lactose intolerant or prefer to limit dairy, you can still follow the Glycemic Diet:

- **Lactose-Free Dairy**: Opt for lactose-free dairy products like lactose-free milk and yogurt.
- **Dairy Alternatives**: Use dairy alternatives like

almond milk, soy yogurt, and coconut milk.

- **Calcium Sources**: Ensure you're getting enough calcium from sources like leafy greens, almonds, and fortified dairy-free products.
- **Lean Proteins**: Rely on lean proteins like poultry, fish, and tofu.
- **Whole Grains**: Incorporate whole grains like oats, quinoa, and rice.

6. Intermittent Fasting and the Glycemic Diet

Intermittent fasting is a popular eating pattern that involves cycling between periods of fasting and eating. You can integrate the principles of the Glycemic Diet into your intermittent fasting routine:

- **Low-GI Meals**: When you do eat, prioritize low-GI foods to help stabilize your blood sugar during the fasting window.

- **Balanced Meals**: Ensure that your meals during eating windows are balanced, including protein, fiber-rich carbohydrates, and healthy fats.

- **Hydration**: Stay well-hydrated, especially during fasting periods.

7. Glycemic Diet for Athletes

Athletes have specific dietary needs. To adapt the Glycemic Diet for athletic performance:

- **Carb Timing**: Prioritize low-GI carbohydrates before and after workouts for sustained energy and glycogen replenishment.
- **Protein**: Include adequate protein to support muscle recovery and growth.

- **Hydration**: Stay well-hydrated, especially during intense training sessions.

- **Snacking**: Plan nutritious, low-GI snacks for sustained energy during longer workouts.

- **Supplements**: Consider supplements like electrolytes and sports drinks as needed for hydration and recovery.

8. Family-Friendly Glycemic Diet

If you're cooking for a family with diverse tastes and dietary needs:

- **Balanced Meals**: Create balanced meals that incorporate a variety of low-GI foods and appeal to different palates.

- **Educate and Involve**: Teach family members about the Glycemic Diet's principles and involve them in meal planning and preparation.

- **Variety**: Embrace variety to keep meals interesting and cater to everyone's preferences.

9. Budget-Friendly Glycemic Diet

Following the Glycemic Diet doesn't have to break the bank. Here are some budget-friendly tips:

- **Seasonal Produce**: Buy fruits and vegetables in season, as they tend to be more affordable.

- **Canned and Frozen**: Consider canned and frozen fruits and vegetables, which are often less expensive and have a longer shelf life.

- **Bulk Purchases**: Buy staples like rice, beans, and oats in bulk to save money in the long run.

- **Cook in Batches**: Prepare meals in larger quantities and freeze portions for later use.

- **Plan and Budget**: Create a meal plan and budget to avoid impulse purchases.

10. Dining Out with the Glycemic Diet

When dining out, you can still adhere to the Glycemic Diet:

- **Check Menus**: Review menus online before going to a restaurant to make informed choices.

- **Ask Questions**: Don't hesitate to ask your server about preparation methods and ingredient substitutions.

- **Share Dishes**: Consider sharing high-GI dishes with dining companions to enjoy a taste without overindulging.

- **Skip Sugary Drinks**: Opt for water or unsweetened beverages instead of sugary sodas or cocktails.

Customizing the Glycemic Diet is all about making it work for you. Tailor it to your dietary preferences,

restrictions, and lifestyle, so it becomes a sustainable and enjoyable way of eating that supports your health and well-being.

Conclusion: Your Glycemic Diet Journey

As we conclude this journey through the Glycemic Diet, remember that it's not just a diet; it's a flexible and adaptable framework for healthy eating. Whether your goal is to manage your weight, control blood sugar, improve heart health, or simply eat better, the Glycemic Diet offers valuable principles that can enhance your overall well-being.

Now, equipped with the knowledge of carbohydrates, the Glycemic Index, and practical strategies, you have the tools to make informed choices about what you eat. You can create balanced, delicious meals that suit your individual needs, preferences, and goals. The Glycemic Diet empowers you to take charge of your health through the food you consume, paving the way for a healthier and more vibrant life.

So, whether you're starting your Glycemic Diet journey or

continuing to refine it, embrace the possibilities, savor the flavors, and relish the nourishment it brings to your body and soul. Your health is your greatest asset, and the Glycemic Diet is here to help you protect and cherish it.

CONCLUSION

In conclusion, the Glycemic Diet is a versatile and adaptable approach to eating that can benefit a wide range of individuals with diverse dietary needs and preferences. Throughout this exploration, we've delved into the fundamental principles of this diet, its applications in weight management, blood sugar control, and heart health, as well as strategies for customizing it to fit your unique lifestyle.

The Glycemic Diet's core concept, the Glycemic Index (GI), ranks carbohydrates based on their effect on blood sugar levels. By emphasizing low-GI foods, this diet promotes stable energy, reduced cravings, and improved overall health. Here are some key takeaways:

1. **Weight Management**: The Glycemic Diet offers a sustainable approach to weight management by focusing on balanced meals, portion control, and reduced cravings for high-GI foods.

2. **Blood Sugar Control**: For individuals with diabetes or prediabetes, this diet can help stabilize blood sugar levels and reduce the risk of complications.

3. **Heart Health**: By supporting blood sugar control, weight management, and improved lipid profiles, the Glycemic Diet can contribute to better heart health and a reduced risk of heart disease.

4. **Customization**: One of the strengths of the Glycemic Diet is its adaptability. You can customize it to align

with various dietary needs and preferences, from vegetarian and vegan diets to gluten-free, paleo, and more.

5. **Practical Strategies**: We've discussed practical strategies for implementing the Glycemic Diet in your daily life, such as choosing whole grains, lean proteins, healthy fats, and fiber-rich foods.

6. **Holistic Approach**: The Glycemic Diet takes a holistic approach to health, considering not only weight and blood sugar but also

overall well-being and long-term health outcomes.

As you embark on your Glycemic Diet journey, keep in mind that it's not just about what you eat; it's about making informed choices that nourish your body, mind, and soul. Whether you're seeking to manage a specific health condition, maintain a healthy weight, or simply eat better, the Glycemic Diet provides a valuable framework for achieving your goals.

So, embrace the possibilities, savor the flavors, and relish the nourishment it brings to your life.

Your health is a lifelong journey, and the Glycemic Diet is a reliable companion along the way, helping you achieve and maintain a balanced, vibrant life through informed choices and sustainable habits.